Mediterranean Diet Cookbook

100+ Fast, Easy, and Delicious Recipes

Michael Scott

Contents

Chapter One

RICE WITH GREENS AND LEMON

20 minutes of preparation time 45 minutes of cooking time 6 people

Difficulty Average in difficulty.

INGREDIENTS:

f 2 cups uncooked long grain rice (soaked in cold water for 20 minutes, then drained) f 3 tablespoons extra virgin olive oil f 1 medium chopped yellow onion 1 minced garlic clove 12 cup orzo pasta f 2 lemons' juice, plus 1 lemon's zest 2 cups low sodium broth f 1 teaspoon salt f 1 good handful chopped parsley 1 tsp. of dill weed

DIRECTIONS:

3 tblsp extra virgin olive oil, heated in a saucepan Stir-fry for 3 to 4 minutes, then add the onions. Toss in the orzo spaghetti with the garlic.

Then add the rice and toss to coat. Add the lemon juice and broth to the pot. Bring to a boil, then reduce to a low heat setting. Cook for 20 minutes with the lid ajar.

Heat should be turned off. Set aside for 10 minutes after covering with plastic wrap. Stir in the lemon zest, dill weed, and parsley after removing the lid. Serve.

(per 100g) nutrition: calorie count: 145 3g Carbohydrates, 9g Fat Protein (three grams) Sodium 893mg

RICE WITH GLACIUM AND HERBS

10 minutes to prepare 30 Minutes of Preparation 4 people

Difficulty Easy difficulty.

INGREDIENTS:\sf 12 cup extra-virgin olive oil 5 minced large garlic cloves 2 cups brown jasmine rice (brown jasmine rice, brown rice, brown rice, brown rice, brown rice, 4 cup hot water 1 tsp. of sea salt 1 tsp. of black pepper 3 tablespoons fresh chopped chives 2 tbsp. chopped parsley 1 tbsp. basil leaves, chopped

DIRECTIONS:

14 cup olive oil, garlic, and rice, combined in a saucepan Heat over medium-low heat, stirring occasionally. Mix in the water, black pepper, and sea salt. Mix everything together one more.

Bring to a boil, then reduce to a low heat setting. Cook, uncovered, for about 30 minutes, stirring periodically.

Mix the remaining 14 cup olive oil with the basil, parsley, and chives until the water is nearly completely absorbed.

Stir until all of the water has been absorbed and the herbs have been well blended.

(per 100g) nutrition: Calories are 304 3g Carbohydrate, 8g Fat Protein (two grams) Sodium 874mg

SALAD WITH MEDIEVAL RICE

10 minutes to prepare 25 minutes of cooking time 4 people

INGREDIENTS: f DIFFICULTY LEVEL: MEDIUM 12 cup extra virgin olive oil 1 cup brown long-grain rice 2 cups hot water a quarter cup of fresh lemon juice 1 minced garlic clove 1 tsp. freshly minced rosemary 1 teaspoon freshly minced mint 3 tblsp. chopped Belgian endives 1 medium-sized chopped red bell pepper 1 chopped hothouse cucumber 12 cup finely chopped green onion 12 cup finely chopped Kalamata olives 14 teaspoon of red pepper flakes feta cheese (crumbled)– 34 cup black pepper, sea salt DIRECTIONS:

In a saucepan on low heat, heat 14 cup olive oil, rice, and a pinch of salt. To coat the rice, stir it in a circular motion. Allow to simmer until all of the water has been absorbed. Occasionally stir the mixture. Fill a large mixing bowl halfway with rice and set aside to cool.

14 cup olive oil, red pepper flakes, olives, green onion, cucumber, bell pepper, endives, mint, rosemary, garlic, and lemon juice in a separate bowl

Toss in the rice and mix well. Mix in the feta cheese with a fork until it is evenly distributed.

Season to taste with salt and pepper. Serve.

(per 100g) nutrition: calorie count: 415 3g Carbohydrates and 34g Fat Protein Content: 7g Sodium 4755mg

SALAD WITH TUNA AND FRESH BEANS

5 minutes of preparation time 20 minutes of cooking time 6 people

Easy to Moderate Difficulty

INGREDIENTS:

f 2 cups f fresh shelled (shucked) beans 2 ft. bay leaves f 3 tablespoons extra-virgin olive oil 1 tbsp. balsamic vinegar black pepper and salt f 1 (6-ounce) can of best-quality tuna f soaked and dried salted capers– 1 tbsp 2 tbsp. parsley, finely minced flat-leaf 1 slice of red onion

DIRECTIONS:

In a saucepan, bring water to a boil with a pinch of salt. Cook for 15 to 20 minutes, or until the beans are tender but firm, after which add the bay leaves and cook for another 15 to

20 minutes. Transfer to a bowl after draining and discarding aromatics.

Dress the beans right away with oil and vinegar. Salt and pepper to taste. Adjust seasoning if necessary. Drain the tuna and toss it into the bean salad in flake form. Combine the capers and parsley in a bowl. Toss well to combine, then top with red onion slices. Serve.

(per 100g) nutrition: calorie count: 85 7g Carbohydrates / 1g Fat Sodium: 863mg/g Protein

CHICKEN PASTA DELICIOUS

10 minutes to prepare 17 minutes of cooking time 4 people

Difficulty Easy difficulty.

INGREDIENTS:

3 skinless, boneless chicken breasts cut into pieces f 9 oz whole-grain pasta f 1/2 cup olives, sliced f 1/2 cup sun-dried tomatoes f 1 tbsp roasted red peppers, chopped f 14 oz can tomato, diced salt and pepper

DIRECTIONS:

Toss everything into the instant pot except the whole-grain pasta.

Cook on high for 12 minutes with the lid closed.

Allow pressure to naturally release once finished. Take the lid off the container.

Stir in the pasta. Re-seal the pot, then set the timer for 5 minutes on the manual setting.

Release the pressure for 5 minutes after completion, then use quick release to release the remaining pressure. Take the lid off the container. Serve after a thorough mix.

(per 100g) nutrition: calorie count: 615 Carbohydrates: 71g, fat: 4g Protein content of 48g Sodium 631mg

RICE BOWL WITH FLAVORS

10 minutes to prepare 14 minutes of cooking time 8 Servings; Moderate Difficulty

INGREDIENTS:

1 pound ground beef f 8 ounces shredded cheddar cheese f 14 ounces canned red beans f 2 ounces taco seasoning f 16 ounces salsa f 2 cups water f 2 cups brown rice f salt and pepper

DIRECTIONS:

Put the instant pot on the sauté setting.

Cook until the meat is brown in the pot.

Stir well to incorporate the water, beans, rice, taco seasoning, pepper, and salt.

Salsa on top Cook on high for 14 minutes with the lid ajar.

When you're finished, quickly release the pressure. Take the lid off the container.

Stir in the cheddar cheese until it has melted completely.

Enjoy your meal!

(per 100g) nutrition: 464 Calories 3 g of fat, 9 g of carbs Protein (two grams) Sodium 612mg

CHEESY MAC AND CHEESE WITH FLAVOR

10 minutes to prepare 10 Minutes of Preparation 6 people

Difficulty Easy difficulty.

INGREDIENTS:

f 16 oz whole-grain elbow pasta f 4 cups water f 1 cup diced canned tomato f 1 tsp garlic, chopped f 2 tbsp olive oil f 1/4 cup green onions, chopped f 1/2 cup parmesan cheese, grated f 1/2 cup mozzarella cheese, grated f 1 cup cheddar cheese, grated f 1/4 cup passata f 1 cup unsweetened almond milk f 1 cup marinated artichoke, diced f

DIRECTIONS:

In a large instant pot, combine the pasta, water, tomatoes, garlic, oil, and salt. Cook on high, covered.

Release pressure for a few minutes after that, then use quick discharge to release the remaining pressure. Take the lid off the container.

Preheat the pot to sauté. Green onion, parmesan cheese, mozzarella cheese, cheddar cheese, passata, almond milk, artichoke, sun-dried tomatoes, and olive are all good additions. Make a thorough mixture.

Cook until the cheese has melted, stirring constantly.

Enjoy your meal!

(per 100g) nutrition: calorie count: 519 5g Carbohydrates 1 g Fat Sodium: 588mg/25g protein

OLIVE RICE WITH CUCUMBER

10 minutes to prepare 10 Minutes of Preparation 8 people

INGREDIENTS: INGREDIENTS: DIFFICULTY LEVEL: MEDIUM

f 2 cups rinsed rice f 1/2 cup pitted olives f 1 cup chopped cucumber f 1 tbsp red wine vinegar f 1 tsp lemon zest, grated f 1 tbsp fresh lemon juice f 2 tbsp olive oil f 2 cups vegetable broth f 1/2 tsp dried oregano f 1 red bell pepper, chopped f 1/2 cup onion, chopped f 1 tbsp olive oil f Pepper f

DIRECTIONS:

Fill the inner pot with oil and set the instant pot to sauté mode. Cook for 3 minutes with the onion. Cook for 1 minute with the bell pepper and oregano.

Stir well to combine the rice and broth. Cook on high for 6 minutes with the lid shut. Allow 10 minutes for pressure to dissipate before utilizing fast release to complete the process. Take the lid off the container.

Mix together the remaining ingredients well. It's ready to eat right away.

(per 100g) nutrition: calorie count: 229 2g Carbohydrates, 1g Fat 210mg Sodium 9g Protein

HERB RESOTTO FLAVORS

10 minutes to prepare 15 minutes of preparation time 4 people

Average Difficulty

INGREDIENTS:

2 cups rice f 2 tbsp grated parmesan cheese f 5 ounces heavy cream f 1 tbsp fresh oregano, chopped f 1 tbsp fresh basil, chopped f 1/2 tbsp sage, chopped f 2 tbsp olive oil f 1 tsp garlic, minced f 4 cups vegetable stock salt and pepper

DIRECTIONS:

Pour oil into the instant pot's inner vessel and set it to sauté mode. In the inner pan of the instant pot, add the garlic and onion and set the pot to sauté. Cook for 2-3 minutes with the garlic and onion.

Stir in the other ingredients, except the parmesan cheese and the heavy cream. Cook for 12 minutes on high, covered.

After that, let the pressure out for 10 minutes before using rapid release to release the rest. Take the lid off the container. Serve with a dollop of cream and some cheese.

(per 100g) nutrition: calorie count: 514 4g Carbohydrates, 6g Fat Protein content: 8g Sodium 488mg

PASTA PREMIUM DELICIOUSNESS

10 minutes to prepare 4 Minutes of Preparation 4 people

Difficulty Easy difficulty.

INGREDIENTS:

8 oz. penne pasta made from whole wheat

1 tbsp lemon juice, freshly squeezed

2 tablespoons chopped fresh parsley

14 oz can chopped tomato 1/4 cup slivered almonds 1/4 cup grated parmesan cheese

prunes (half cup)

1/2 cup sliced zucchini 1/2 cup chopped asparagus

1 3/4 cup vegetable stock 1/2 cup carrots 1/2 cup broccoli, chopped

salt with pepper

1. In a large instant pot, combine the stock, parsley, tomatoes, prunes, zucchini, asparagus, carrots, and broccoli.

well. Cook for 4 minutes on high, covered. When you're finished, quickly remove the pressure. Remove the lid from the container. Serve after thoroughly combining the remaining ingredients.

(per 100g) nutrition: Calorie count: 303 5g Carbohydrates 6g Fat Protein content: 8g Sodium 918mg

Preparation Time: 10 Minutes ROASTED PEPPER PASTA 13 minutes of cooking time 6 people

INGREDIENTS: INGREDIENTS: DIFFICULTY LEVEL: MEDIUM

1 pound whole wheat penne pasta, 1 tablespoon Italian spice 1 cup feta cheese, crumbled f 1 tbsp olive oil f 4 cups vegetable broth f 1 tbsp garlic, minced f 1/2 onion, chopped f 14 oz jar roasted red peppers f 1 cup feta cheese, crumbled salt and pepper

DIRECTIONS:

Blend the roasted peppers until smooth in the blender. Fill the inner pot of the instant pot halfway with oil and set aside.

Place the jug in the sauté position. Set the Instant Pot to sauté and add the garlic and onion to the inner cup. Cook for 2-3 minutes with the garlic and onion.

Cook for 2 minutes with the mixed roasted pepper.

Stir in the other ingredients, except the feta cheese. Cook for 8 minutes on high with the lid tightly closed. When you're finished, let the pressure out naturally for 5 minutes before employing rapid release to get the last of it out. Take the lid off the container. Serve garnished with feta cheese.

(per 100g) nutrition: calorie count: 459 6 g Carbohydrates 1 g Fat Protein (three grams) Sodium 724 mg

TOMATO RICE WITH CHEESE BASIL

10 minutes to prepare 26-minute cooking time 8 people

INGREDIENTS: INGREDIENTS: DIFFICULTY LEVEL: MEDIUM

1 1/2 cups brown rice f 1 cup grated parmesan cheese f 1/4 cup chopped fresh basil f 2 cups halved grape tomatoes f 8 oz can tomato sauce f 1 3/4 cup vegetable broth f 1 tbsp garlic f 1/2 cup diced onion f 1 tbsp olive oil salt and pepper

DIRECTIONS:

Pour oil into the instant pot's inner basin and set it to sauté. Set the inner vessel of the instant pot on sauté mode and add the garlic and onion. Sauté for 4 minutes after adding garlic and onion. Stir thoroughly to include the rice, tomato sauce, stock, pepper, and salt.

Cook for 22 minutes on high, sealed.

Allow 10 minutes for pressure to relax before using rapid release to release the remainder. Cap should be removed. In a mixing bowl, combine the remaining ingredients. Enjoy your meal!

(per 100g) nutrition: calorie count: 208 6 g Carbohydrates 1 g Fat Protein (three grams) Sodium 863mg

MAC & CHEESE is a dish that combines the flavors of macaroni and cheese

10 minutes to prepare 4 Minutes of Preparation 8 people

Difficulty Easy difficulty.

INGREDIENTS:

l 1 pound whole grain pasta l 1/2 cup grated parmesan cheese l 4 cups shredded cheddar cheese l 1 cup milk l 1/4 teaspoon garlic powder l 1/2 teaspoon ground mustard l 2 tablespoons olive oil l 4 cups water

DIRECTIONS:

1. Fill the instant pot halfway with water and add the pasta, garlic powder, mustard, oil, pepper, and salt. Cook on high for 4 minutes with a tightly sealed bag. When you're finished, quickly remove the pressure. Lid must be removed. Serve with the remaining ingredients, which have been well mixed.

509 calories per 100g 8g Carbohydrates, 7g Fat Protein (three grams) Sodium 766 mg

TUNA PASTA is a type of pasta that is made from tuna.

10 minutes to prepare 8-Minute Preparation Difficulty: 6 Serves Average in difficulty.

INGREDIENTS:

I 10 oz tuna can, drained I 15 oz whole wheat rotini pasta I 4 oz mozzarella cheese, cubed I 1/2 cup parmesan cheese, grated I 1 tsp dried basil I 14 oz can tomato I 4 cups vegetable broth I 1 tbsp garlic, minced I 8 oz mushrooms, sliced I 2 zucchinis, sliced I 1 onion, chopped

DIRECTIONS:

Fill the inner pot of the instant pot halfway with oil and set the pot to sauté. Sauté until the onion is softened, then add the mushrooms, zucchini, and onion. Sauté for a minute with the garlic.

In a large mixing bowl, combine the pasta, basil, tuna, tomatoes, and broth. Cook for 4 minutes on high, sealed.

Release pressure for 5 minutes after it's finished, then use quick release to release the remaining pressure. Take the lid off the container. Serve with the remaining ingredients, which have been thoroughly mixed in.

(per 100g) nutrition: calorie count: 346 3g Carbohydrates, 9g Fat Protein (three grams) Sodium 830mg

PANINI WITH MIXED AVOCADO AND TURKEY

5 minutes of preparation time 8-Minute Preparation 2 people

Difficulty Easy difficulty.

INGREDIENTS:

14 lb. thinly sliced mesquite smoked turkey breast f 1 cup whole fresh spinach leaves, divided f 2 slices provolone cheese f 1 tablespoon olive oil, divided f 2 ciabatta rolls

12 ripe avocado (14) cup mayonnaise DIRECTIONS:

Combine mayonnaise and avocado in a mixing bowl and thoroughly combine. The Panini press should then be preheated.

halve the bread rolls and brush the insides with olive oil. Then layer provolone, turkey breast, roasted red pepper, spinach leaves, and avocado mixture before covering with the other bread slice.

Place the sandwich in the Panini press and cook for 5 to 8 minutes, or until the cheese has melted and the bread is crisp and ridged.

(per 100g) nutrition: calorie count: 546 Carbohydrates: 9 g (8 g fat) Protein content: 8g Sodium 582mg

MANGO WRAP WITH CUCUMBER AND CHICKEN

5 minutes of preparation time 20 minutes of cooking time 1 portion

INGREDIENTS: Difficult DIFFICULTY LEVEL: DIFFICULT DIFFICULTY LEVEL: DIFFICULT DIFFICULTY LE

12 medium cucumbers, cut lengthwise f 12 ripe mangos f 1 tbsp salad dressing of choice f 1 whole wheat tortilla wrap f 1-inch thick slice of chicken breast, around 6-inch in length f 2 tbsp oil for frying f 2 tbsp whole wheat flour f 2 to 4 lettuce leaves to taste with salt and pepper

DIRECTIONS:

Cook a total of 6 inch strips from a chicken breast that has been sliced into 1-inch strips. It'd be the equivalent of two chicken strips. Keep any leftover chicken in the fridge for later.

Pepper and salt the chicken. Using whole wheat flour as a dredging agent, coat the chicken in it.

Place a small nonstick fry pan over medium heat to heat the oil. When the oil is hot, add the chicken strips and cook for 5 minutes per side, or until golden brown.

Cook tortilla wraps for 3 to 5 minutes in the oven while the chicken is cooking. Place on a plate and set aside.

Only use 12 of the cucumber after slicing it lengthwise. Remove the pith from a cucumber by peeling it and cutting it into quarters. Place the two cucumber slices 1 inch from the edge of the tortilla wrap.

Half of the mango should be sliced and the other half should be stored with the seeds. Remove the seeds from the mango and slice it into strips to go on top of the cucumber on the tortilla wrap.

When the chicken is done, arrange it in a line next to the cucumber.

Drizzle salad dressing of choice over cucumber leaf.

Serve the tortilla wrap and take a bite.

(per 100g) nutrition: Calories: 434 65g Carbohydrates/10g Fat Protein (21g) Sodium: 691 mg

BREAD FROM THE MIDDLE EAST WITH FATTOUSH

10 minutes to prepare 15 minutes of preparation time 6 people

Level of Difficulty: Difficult

INGREDIENTS: f 2 pita bread loaves f 1 tbsp Extra Virgin Olive Oil f 1/2 tsp sumac (reserve some for later) 2 cups chopped fresh parsley leaves f 1 cup chopped fresh mint leaves f 1 heart of Romaine lettuce f 1 English cucumber f 5 Roma tomatoes f 5 green onions f 5 radishes f 2 cups chopped fresh parsley leaves f 2 cups chopped fresh parsley leaves f 1 cup chopped fresh mint leaves f Dressing 1 1/2 lime, lime juice f 1/3 cup Extra Virgin Olive Oil f 1 teaspoon ground sumac f 1/4 teaspoon ground cinnamon f scant 1/4 teaspoon ground allspice

DIRECTIONS:

1. Toast the pita bread in the toaster oven for 5 minutes. The pita bread should then be broken into pieces. 2. Heat 3 tbsp olive oil in a large pan over medium heat for 3 minutes. Fry the pita bread until golden brown.

4 minutes while tossing around until browned

Season with salt, pepper, and 1/2 teaspoon sumac. Remove the pita chips from the heat and drain on paper towels.

In a large salad bowl, combine the chopped lettuce, cucumber, tomatoes, green onions, sliced radish, mint leaves, and parsley.

In a small bowl, whisk together all of the ingredients for the lime vinaigrette.

Toss the salad with the dressing and toss well. Add the pita bread to the mix.

Enjoy your meal!

(per 100g) nutrition: Calories: 192 8 g of fat Carbohydrates (1 g) Protein: 9 g Sodium: 655 mg

GLUTEN-FREE FOCACCIA WITH GARLIC & TOMATO

5 minutes of preparation time 20 minutes of cooking time 8 people

Difficulty INGREDIENTS: INGREDIENTS: DIFFICULTY LEVEL: DIFFICULTY LEVEL: DIFFIC

f 1 egg f 12 tsp lemon juice f 1 tbsp honey f 4 tbsp olive oil f A pinch of sugar f 1 14 cup warm water f 1 tbsp active dry yeast f 2 tsp rosemary, chopped f 2 tsp thyme, chopped f 2 tsp basil, chopped f 2 garlic cloves, minced f 1 14 tsp sea salt f 2 t For dusting, use gluten-free cornmeal

DIRECTIONS:

Turn the oven on for 5 minutes and then off, keeping the oven door closed.

Warm water and a pinch of sugar are combined in a mixing bowl. Swirl in the yeast. Allow 7 minutes for this process.

Herbs, garlic, salt, xanthan gum, starch, and flours should all be combined in a large mixing bowl. Pour the yeast into the flours once it has finished proofing. Egg, lemon juice, honey, and olive oil are all whisked together.

Mix thoroughly and bake in a cornmeal-dusted square pan that has been well-greased. Fresh garlic, additional herbs, and sliced tomatoes can be added to the top. Allow to rise for half an hour in a preheated oven.

Preheat the oven to 375 degrees Fahrenheit and cook for 20 minutes after it has been preheated. Once the tops are lightly browned, the focaccia is ready. Remove the pan and oven from the heat as soon as possible. Warm is best. (per 100g) nutrition: calorie count: 251 4g Carbohydrates, 9g Fat Protein (four grams) Sodium (366mg)

MUSHROOM BURGERS GRILLED

15 minutes for preparation 10 Minutes of Preparation 4 people

Difficulty Average in difficulty.

INGREDIENTS:

f 2 Bibb lettuce leaves, halved f 4 red onion slices f 4 tomato slices f 4 whole wheat buns, toasted f 2 tbsp olive oil f 14 tsp cayenne pepper, optional f 1 garlic clove, minced f 1 tbsp sugar f 12 cup water f 1/3 cup balsamic vinegar f 4 large Portobello mushroom caps, around 5-inches in diameter

DIRECTIONS:

Clean the mushrooms with a damp cloth after removing the stems. Place the fish gill-side up in a baking dish.

Combine olive oil, cayenne pepper, garlic, sugar, water, and vinegar in a mixing bowl and thoroughly combine. Pour over the mushrooms and set aside for at least an hour to marinate.

Preheat the grill to medium high and grease the grill grate when the hour is nearly up.

5 minutes per side on the grill, or until tender. To keep the marinade from drying out, baste the mushrooms with it.

Place 12 of the bread buns on a plate and top with a slice of onion, mushroom, tomato, and one lettuce leaf to assemble. Cover the top half of the bun with the remaining bun half. Serve and enjoy the rest of the ingredients.

(per 100g) nutrition: calorie count: 244 Carbohydrates: 32 g fat 3 g fat Protein (1 gram) Sodium 693mg

BABA GHANOUSH OF THE MEDIEVAL

10 minutes to prepare 25 minutes of cooking time 4 people

INGREDIENTS: INGREDIENTS: DIFFICULTY LEVEL: MEDIUM

2 eggplants, sliced lengthwise f 2 rounds of flatbread or pita f 1 bulb garlic f 1 red bell pepper, halved and seeded f 1 tbsp chopped fresh basil f 1 tbsp olive oil f 1 tsp black pepper f DIRECTIONS:

Preheat the grill to medium high and coat the grate with cooking spray.

Wrap foil around the tops of the garlic bulbs. Cook for at least 20 minutes on the cooler side of the grill. On the hottest part of the grill, place the bell pepper and eggplant slices. Both sides should be cooked.

After the bulbs have finished cooking, remove the skins from the roasted garlic and place it in a food processor. Combine the olive oil, pepper, basil, lemon juice, grilled red bell pepper, and grilled eggplant in a large mixing bowl. Pour into a bowl after pureeing.

To warm the bread, grill each side for at least 30 seconds. Enjoy with bread and pureed dip.

(per 100g) nutrition: calorie count: 6 3g Carbohydrates 8g Fat Protein (three grams) Sodium 593mg

DINNER ROLLS WITH MULTI GRAINS & NO GLUTEN

10 minutes to prepare 20 minutes of cooking time 8 people

Difficulty Average in difficulty.

INGREDIENTS:

12 cup tapioca starch f 14 cup brown teff flour f 14 cup flax meal f 14 cup amaranth flour f 14 cup sorghum flour f 34 cup brown rice flour f 12 tsp apple cider vinegar f 3 tbsp olive oil f

2 eggs f 1 tsp baking powder f 1 tsp salt f 2 tsp xanthan gum
DIRECTIONS:

In a small mixing bowl, combine the water, honey, and yeast. Allow 10 minutes to pass.

Baking powder, salt, xanthan gum, flax meal, sorghum flour, teff flour, tapioca starch, amaranth flour, and brown rice flour should all be mixed together with a paddle mixer.

Whisk vinegar, olive oil, and eggs together in a medium bowl.

Pour vinegar and yeast mixture into dry ingredients bowl and stir to combine.

Using cooking spray, spray a 12-muffin tin. Fill 12 muffin tins evenly with dough and set aside to rise for an hour.

Preheat the oven to 375 degrees Fahrenheit and bake the dinner rolls for about 20 minutes, or until golden brown on top.

Take the dinner rolls and muffin tins out of the oven as soon as possible and set them aside to cool.

Warm is best.

(per 100g) nutrition: Calorie count: 207 8g Carbohydrates, 3g Fat 6 oz. Sodium 844mg

Chapter Two

MUFFINS QUINOA PIZZA

15 minutes for preparation 30 Minutes of Preparation 4 people

Difficulty Easy difficulty.

INGREDIENTS:

f 1 cup uncooked quinoa f 2 large eggs f 12 medium diced onion f 1 cup diced bell pepper f 1 cup shredded mozzarella cheese f 1 tbsp dried basil f 1 tbsp dried oregano f 2 tsp garlic powder f 1/8 tsp salt f 1 tsp crushed red peppers f 12 cup roasted red pepper, chopped* DIRECTIONS:

Preheat the oven to 350 degrees Fahrenheit (180 degrees Celsius). Follow the package directions for cooking the quinoa. In a mixing bowl, mix together all of the ingredients (except the sauce). All ingredients should be thoroughly combined.

Fill muffin tins evenly with quinoa pizza mixture. 12 muffins are made from this recipe. Bake for 30 minutes, or until golden brown and crisp around the edges.

Enjoy 1 or 2 tablespoons of pizza sauce on top!

(per 100g) nutrition: Calorie count: 303 3g Carbohydrates, 1g Fat Protein Content: 21g Sodium 694mg

BREAD WITH ROSEMARY AND WALNUT

5 minutes of preparation time 45 minutes of cooking time Difficulty: 8 servings Difficulty level:

INGREDIENTS:

12 cup chopped walnuts f 4 tbsp fresh, chopped rosemary f 1 1/3 cups lukewarm carbonated water f 1 tbsp honey f 12 cup extra virgin olive oil f 1 tsp apple cider vinegar f 3 eggs f 5 tsp instant dry yeast granules f 1 tsp salt f 1 tbsp xanthan gum f 14 cup buttermilk powder

DIRECTIONS:

Whisk eggs vigorously in a large mixing bowl. 1 cup warm water, 1 tablespoon honey, 1 tablespoon olive oil, and 1 tablespoon vinegar

Except for the rosemary and walnuts, continue to beat while adding the remaining ingredients.

Keep pounding away. Stir in a small amount of warm water if the dough is too stiff. Shaggy and thick dough is ideal.

Continue kneading until the rosemary and walnuts are evenly distributed.

Allow dough to rise for 30 minutes by covering it with a clean towel and placing it in a warm place.

Preheat the oven to 400oF 15 minutes into the rising time.

Preheat a 2-quart Dutch oven without the lid by liberally greasing it with olive oil.

Remove the pot from the oven and place the dough inside once it has finished rising. Spread the dough evenly in the pot using a wet spatula.

Brush 2 tbsp olive oil on the tops of the bread slices, cover Dutch oven, and bake for 35 to 45 minutes. Remove the baked bread from the oven when it is done. Remove the bread from the pot carefully. Before slicing, let the bread cool for at least ten minutes. Enjoy your meal!

(per 100g) nutrition: calorie count: 424 Carbohydrates: 19 g fat, 19 g sugar Protein Content: 7g Sodium 844mg

YUM YUM YUM YUM YUM YUM YUM YUM YUC

5 minutes of preparation time 10 Minutes of Preparation 4 people

Difficulty Easy difficulty.

INGREDIENTS:

12 cup celery f 14 cup green onion chopped f 1 tsp Worcestershire sauce f 1 tsp lemon juice f 1 tbsp Dijon mustard f 12 cup light mayonnaise f 1 pound shrimp crab

DIRECTIONS:

Celery, onion, Worcestershire, lemon juice, mustard, and mayonnaise should all be thoroughly combined in a medium bowl. Pepper and salt to taste. The almonds and crabs should be added last.

Apply olive oil to the sliced sides of the bread and smear the crab mixture on top before covering with another slice of bread.

In a Panini press, cook the sandwich until the bread is crisp and ridged.

(per 100g) nutrition: calorie count: 248 12 g Carbohydrates 9 g Fat Protein (five grams) Sodium 845mg

PERFECT PIZZA & PASTRY

Preparation Time : 35 minutes 15 minutes of preparation time Servings : 10

Level of Difficulty: Moderate

INGREDIENTS:

For the Pizza Dough:

f 2-tsp honey f 1/4-oz. active dry yeast f 11/4-cups warm water (about 120 °F) f 2-tbsp olive oil f 1-tsp sea salt f 3-cups whole grain flour + 1/4-cup, as needed for rolling f For the Pizza Topping:

f 1-cup pesto sauce f 1-cup artichoke hearts f 1-cup wilted spinach leaves f 1-cup sun-dried tomato f 1/2-cup Kalamata olives f 4-oz. feta cheese f 4-oz. mixed cheese of equal parts low-fat mozzarella, asiago, and provolone Olive oil Optional Topping Add-Ons: f Bell pepper f Chicken breast, strips Fresh basil f Pine nuts

DIRECTIONS: For the Pizza Dough:

Preheat your oven to 350 °F.

Stir the honey and yeast with the warm water in your food processor with a dough attachment.

Blend the

mixture until fully combined. Let the mixture to rest for 5 minutes to ensure the activity of the yeast through the appearance of bubbles on the surface.

Pour in the olive oil. Add the salt, and blend for half a minute. Add gradually 3 cups of flour, about half a cup at a time, blending for a couple of minutes between each addition.

Let your processor knead the mixture for 10 minutes until smooth and elastic, sprinkling it with flour whenever necessary to prevent the dough from sticking to the processor bowl's surfaces.

Take the dough from the bowl. Let it stand for 15 minutes, covered with a moist, warm towel.

Roll out the dough to a half-inch thickness, dusting it with flour as needed. Poke holes indiscriminately on the dough using a fork to prevent crust bubbling. Place the perforated, rolled dough on a pizza stone or baking sheet. Bake for 5 minutes.

For the Pizza Topping:

Lightly brush the baked pizza shell with olive oil.

Pour over the pesto sauce and spread thoroughly over the pizza shell's surface, leaving out a half-inch space around its edge as the crust.

Top the pizza with artichoke hearts, wilted spinach leaves, sun-dried tomatoes, and olives. (Top with more add-ons, as desired.) Cover the top with the cheese.

Put the pizza directly to the oven rack. Bake for 10 minutes until the cheese is bubbling and melting from the center to the end. Let the pizza chill for 5 minutes before slicing.

(per 100g) nutrition: 8 Calories 1g Fats 7g Carbohydrates Protein (1 gram) 942mg Sodium

MARGHERITA MEDITERRANEAN MODEL

15 minutes for preparation 15 minutes of preparation time Servings : 10

Level of Difficulty: Moderate

INGREDIENTS:

f 1-batch pizza shell f 2-tbsp olive oil f 1/2-cup crushed tomatoes f 3-Roma tomatoes, sliced 1/4-inch thick f 1/2-cup fresh basil leaves, thinly sliced f 6-oz. block mozzarella, cut into 1/4-inch slices, blot-dry with a paper towel f 1/2-tsp sea salt

DIRECTIONS:

Preheat your oven to 450 °F.

Lightly brush the pizza shell with olive oil. Thoroughly spread the crushed tomatoes over the pizza shell,

leaving a half-inch space around its edge as the crust.

Top the pizza with the Roma tomato slices, basil leaves, and mozzarella slices. Sprinkle salt over the pizza.

Transfer the pizza directly on the oven rack. Bake until the cheese melts from the center to the crust. Set aside before slicing.

(per 100g) nutrition: calorie count: 251 Fats (8g) 34g Carbohydrates 9g Protein 844mg Sodium

PORTABLE PACKED PICNIC PIECES

5 minutes of preparation time Cooking Time : 0 minutes Servings : 1 Difficulty Easy difficulty.

INGREDIENTS:

f 1-slice of whole-wheat bread, cut into bite-size pieces

f 10-pcs cherry tomatoes

f 1/4-oz. aged cheese, sliced f 6-pcs oil-cured olives
DIRECTIONS:

1. Pack each of the ingredients in a portable container to serve you while snacking on the go.

(per 100g) nutrition: 197 Calories 9g Fats 22g Carbohydrates Protein Content: 7g 499mg Sodium

FRITTATA FILLED WITH ZESTY ZUCCHINI & TOMATO TOPPINGS

10 minutes to prepare 15 minutes of preparation time 4 people

Difficulty Easy difficulty.

INGREDIENTS:

f 8-pcs eggs f 1/4-tsp red pepper, crushed f 1/4-tsp salt f 1-tbsp olive oil f 1-pc small zucchini, sliced thinly lengthwise f 1/2-cup red or yellow cherry tomatoes, halved f 1/3 -cup walnuts, coarsely chopped f 2-oz. bite-sized fresh mozzarella balls (bocconcini)

DIRECTIONS:

Preheat your broiler. Meanwhile, whisk together the eggs, crushed red pepper, and salt in a mediumsized bowl. Set aside.

In a 10-inch broiler-proof skillet placed over medium-high heat, heat the olive oil. Arrange the slices of zucchini in an even layer on the bottom of the skillet. Cook for 3 minutes, turning them once, halfway through.

Top the zucchini layer with cherry tomatoes. Fill the egg mixture over vegetables in skillet. Top with walnuts and mozzarella balls.

Switch to medium heat. Cook until the sides begin to set. By using a spatula, lift the frittata for the uncooked portions of the egg mixture to flow underneath.

Place the skillet on the broiler. Broil the frittata 4-inches from the heat for 5 minutes until the top is set. To serve, cut the frittata into wedges.

Nutrition (for 100g): 284 Calories 14g Fats 4g Carbohydrates 17g Protein 788mg Sodium

BANANA SOUR CREAM BREAD

10 minutes to prepare Cooking Time : 1 hour 10 minutes Servings : 32

INGREDIENTS: INGREDIENTS: DIFFICULTY LEVEL: MEDIUM

f White sugar (.25 cup)

f Cinnamon (1 tsp.+ 2 tsp.)

f Butter (.75)

f White sugar (3 cups)

f Eggs (3)

f Very ripe bananas, mashed (6) f Sour cream (16 oz. container)
f Vanilla extract (2 tsp.)

f Salt (.5 tsp.)

f Baking soda (3 tsp.)

f All-purpose flour (5 cups)

f Optional: Chopped walnuts (1 cup)

f Also Needed: 4 - 7 by 3-inch loaf pans

DIRECTIONS:

Set the oven to reach 300°Fahrenheit. Grease the loaf pans.

Sift the sugar and one teaspoon of the cinnamon. Dust the pan with the mixture.

Cream the butter with the rest of the sugar. Mash the bananas with the eggs, cinnamon, vanilla, sour

cream, salt, baking soda, and the flour. Toss in the nuts last.

Dump the mixture into the pans. Bake it for one hour. Serve Nutrition (for 100g): 263 Calories 4g Fat 9g Carbohydrates 7g Protein 633mg Sodium

Chapter Three

HOMEMADE PITA BREAD

15 minutes for preparation

Cooking Time : 5 hours (includes rising times)

Servings : 7

INGREDIENTS: Difficult DIFFICULTY LEVEL: DIFFICULT DIFFICULTY LEVEL: DIFFICULT DIFFICULTY LE

f Dried yeast (.25 oz.)

f Sugar (.5 tsp.)

f Bread flour /mixture of all-purpose & whole wheat (5 cups + more for dusting)

f Salt (.5 tsp.)

f Water (.25 cup or as needed) f Oil as needed DIRECTIONS:

Dissolve the yeast and sugar in ¼ of a cup lukewarm water in a small mixing container. Wait for about 15 minutes (ready when it's frothy).

In another container, sift the flour and salt. Make a hole in the center and add the yeast mixture (+) one cup of water. Knead the dough.

Situate it onto a lightly floured surface and knead.

Put a drop of oil into the bottom of a large bowl and roll the dough in it to cover the surface.

Place a dampened tea towel over the container of dough. Wrap the bowl with a damp cloth and place it in a warm spot for at least two hours or overnight. (The dough will double its size).

Punch the dough down and knead the bread and divide it into small balls. Flatten the balls into thick oval discs.

Dust a tea towel using the flour and place the oval discs on top, leaving enough room to expand between them. Powder with flour and lay another clean cloth on top. Let it rise for another one to two hours.

Set the oven at 425° Fahrenheit. Situate several baking sheets in the oven to heat briefly. Lightly grease the warmed baking sheets with oil and place the oval bread discs on them.

Sprinkle the ovals lightly with water, and bake until they are lightly browned or for six to eight minutes.

Serve them while they are warm. Arrange the flatbread on a wire rack and wrap them in a clean, dry cloth to keep soft for later.

(per 100g) nutrition: 210 Calories 4g Fat 6g Carbohydrates 6 oz. 881mg Sodium

FLATBREAD SANDWICHES

10 minutes to prepare 20 minutes of cooking time 6 people

Difficulty Easy difficulty.

INGREDIENTS:

f Olive oil (1 tbsp.)

f 7-Grain pilaf (5 oz. pkg.)

f English seedless cucumber (1 cup) f Seeded tomato (1 cup)

f Crumbled feta cheese (.25 cup)

f Fresh lemon juice (2 tbsp.)

f Freshly cracked black pepper (.25 tsp.)

f Plain hummus (7 oz. container) f Whole grain white flatbread wraps (3 @ 8 oz. each)

DIRECTIONS:

Cook the pilaf as directed on the package instructions and cool.

Chop and combine the tomato, cucumber, cheese, oil, pepper, and lemon juice. Fold in the pilaf.

Prepare the wraps with the hummus on one side. Spoon in the pilaf and fold.

Slice into a sandwich and serve.

(per 100g) nutrition: 310 Calories 9g Fat 8g Carbohydrates 10g Protein 745mg Sodium

CHICKEN WITH CAPER SAUCE

10 minutes to prepare Cooking Time : 18 minutes Servings : 5

Level of Difficulty: Moderate

INGREDIENTS:

For Chicken:

f 2 eggs f Salt and ground black pepper, as required

f 1 cup dry breadcrumbs

f 2 tablespoons olive oil f 1½ pounds skinless, boneless chicken breast halves, pounded into ¾inch thickness and cut into pieces For Capers Sauce:

f 3 tablespoons capers

f ½ cup dry white wine

f 3 tablespoons fresh lemon juice

f Salt and ground black pepper, as required f 2 tablespoons fresh parsley, chopped DIRECTIONS: For chicken: in a shallow dish, add the eggs, salt and black pepper and beat until well combined. In another shallow dish, place breadcrumbs. Soak the chicken pieces in egg mixture then coat with the breadcrumbs evenly. Shake off the excess breadcrumbs.

Cook the oil over medium heat and cook the chicken pieces for about 5-7 minutes per side or until desired doneness. With a slotted spoon, situate the chicken pieces onto a paper towel lined plate. With a piece of the foil, cover the chicken pieces to keep them warm.

In the same skillet, incorporate all the sauce ingredients except parsley and cook for about 2-3 minutes, stirring continuously. Mix in the parsley and remove from heat. Serve the chicken pieces with the topping of capers sauce.

Nutrition (for 100g): 352 Calories 5g Fat 9g Carbohydrates Protein (two grams) 741mg Sodium

TURKEY BURGERS WITH MANGO SALSA

15 minutes for preparation 10 Minutes of Preparation Difficulty: 6 Serves Easy difficulty.

INGREDIENTS:

f 1½ pounds ground turkey breast f 1 teaspoon sea salt, divided f ¼ teaspoon freshly ground black pepper f 2 tablespoons extra-virgin olive oil f 2 mangos, peeled, pitted, and cubed f ½ red onion, finely chopped f Juice of 1 lime f 1 garlic clove, minced f ½ jalapeño pepper, seeded and finely minced f 2 tablespoons chopped fresh cilantro leaves

DIRECTIONS:

1. Form the turkey breast into 4 patties and season with ½ teaspoon of sea salt and the pepper. Cook the olive oil in a nonstick skillet until it shimmers. Add the turkey patties and cook for about 5 minutes per side until browned. While the patties cook, mix the mango, red onion, lime juice, garlic, jalapeño, cilantro, and remaining ½ teaspoon of sea salt in a small bowl. Spoon the salsa over the turkey patties and serve.

Nutrition (for 100g): 384 Calories 3g Fat 27g Carbohydrates 34g Protein 692mg Sodium

15-MINUTE HERB-ROASTED TURKEY BREAST

Time to Cook: 112 hours

6 Servings

INGREDIENTS: INGREDIENTS: INGREDIENTS: INGREDIENTS: INGREDIENTS:

f f 2 tbsp extra-virgin olive oil 4 minced garlic cloves f 1 tablespoon chopped fresh thyme leaves f 1 tablespoon chopped fresh rosemary leaves f 1 tablespoon lemon zest 2 tblsp fresh Italian parsley leaves, chopped 1 (6-pound) bone-in, skin-on turkey breast f 1 teaspoon ground mustard f 1 teaspoon sea salt f 14 teaspoon freshly ground black pepper f 1 cup white wine, dry

DIRECTIONS:

Preheat oven to 325 degrees Fahrenheit. Combine the olive oil, garlic, lemon zest, thyme, rosemary, parsley, mustard, salt, and pepper in a large mixing bowl. Brush the herb mixture evenly over the turkey breast's surface, and loosen and rub the skin underneath. Place the skin-side up turkey breast in a roasting pan on a rack.

In the pan, pour the wine. Roast for 1 to 112 hours, or until the turkey reaches a temperature of 165 degrees F on the inside. Remove from the oven and set aside for 20 minutes before carving, tented with aluminum foil to keep warm.

Calories per 100g: 392 2g Carbohydrates/1g Fat 84 grams of protein 741 milligrams sodium

SAUSAGE OF CHICKEN AND PEPPERS

Time to Prepare: 10 minutes Time to cook: 20 minutes 6 Servings

Level of Difficulty: Moderate

INGREDIENTS:

f 6 Italian chicken sausage links 2 tablespoons extra-virgin olive oil 12 cup dry white wine f 12 teaspoon sea salt f 14 teaspoon freshly ground black pepper f Pinch red pepper flakes DIRECTIONS:

1. Heat the olive oil in a large skillet over medium heat until it shimmers. Cook for 5 to 7 minutes, turning occasionally, until browned and internal temperature reaches 165°F. Remove the sausage from the pan with tongs and place it on a platter tented with aluminum foil to keep it warm. 2. Add the onion, red bell pepper, and green bell pepper to the skillet and return it to the heat. Cook, stirring occasionally, until the vegetables are browning. Stir in the garlic for 30 seconds.

continuously.

3. Combine the wine, sea salt, pepper, and red pepper flakes in a mixing bowl. Any browned bits from the bottom of the pan should be pulled out and folded in. Cook for another 4 minutes, stirring occasionally, until the liquid has reduced by half.

Serve the sausages with the peppers on top.

Nutritional Information (per 100g): Calories 173 6g Carbohydrates 1g Fat 582mg Sodium 22g Protein

PICCATA WITH CHICKEN

Time to Prepare: 10 minutes Time to prepare: 15 minutes 6 Servings

INGREDIENTS: INGREDIENTS: INGREDIENTS: INGREDIENTS: INGREDIENTS:

12 cup whole-wheat flour 12 teaspoon sea salt 1/8 teaspoon freshly ground black pepper 112 pound chicken breasts, cut into 6 pieces f 3 tablespoons extra-virgin olive oil 1 cup unsalted chicken broth 12 cup dry white wine 1 lemon juice f 1 lemon zest f 14 cup drained and rinsed capers f 14 cup chopped fresh parsley leaves

DIRECTIONS:

Whisk together the flour, sea salt, and pepper in a shallow dish. Using a pastry brush, coat the chicken in flour and tap off any excess. Heat the olive oil until it begins to shimmer.

Cook for about 4 minutes per side until the chicken is browned. Remove the chicken from the pan and cover with aluminum foil to keep it warm.

Reheat the skillet and add the broth, wine, lemon juice, lemon zest, and capers. Scoop any browned bits from the pan's bottom with the back of a spoon and fold them in. Continue to cook until the liquid has thickened. Remove the chicken from the pan and return it to the skillet. Toss in the coat. Serve with parsley on top.

Nutritional Information (per 100g): Calories 153 9 g Carbohydrates 2 g Fat 692mg sodium, 8g protein

TUSCAN CHICKEN IN A SINGLE PAN

Time to Prepare: 10 minutes Time to cook: 25 minutes 6 Servings

Level of Difficulty: Difficulty

INGREDIENTS:

1 pound boneless, skinless chicken breasts, cut into 34-inch pieces f 1 onion, chopped f 1 red bell pepper, chopped f 3 garlic cloves, minced f 12 cup dry white wine, divided

f 1 tablespoon dried Italian seasoning f 12 teaspoon sea salt f 1/8 teaspoon freshly ground black pepper f 1/8 teaspoon red pepper flakes f 14 cup chopped fresh basil leaves f 1 (14-ounce) can crushed tomatoes, undrained f 1 (14-ounce) can chopped tomatoes, drained f 1 (14-ounce) can white beans, drained f 1 tablespoon dried Italian seasoning f 12 teaspoon sea salt f 1/8 teaspoon freshly ground black pepper f 1/8 teaspoon red

1. Heat 2 tablespoons olive oil until it shimmers. Cook until the chicken is browned.

Remove

Remove the chicken from the skillet and place it on a platter, tented with foil to keep it warm. 2. Return the skillet to the heat and add the remaining olive oil to it. Combine the onion and red bell pepper in a large mixing bowl. Cook, stirring occasionally, until the vegetables are soft. Cook for 30 seconds, stirring constantly.

Stir in the wine, and scrape any browned bits from the bottom of the pan with the back of a spoon.

Cook for 1 minute, stirring constantly.

Combine the crushed and chopped tomatoes, white beans, Italian seasoning, sea salt, pepper, and red pepper flakes in a large mixing bowl. Allow to simmer for a while. Cook, stirring occasionally for 5 minutes.

Return the chicken to the skillet, along with any accumulated juices. Cook until the chicken is fully cooked. Remove from the heat and add the basil just before serving.

Nutritional Information (per 100g): Calories 271 8 g fat, 29 g carbs Protein: 14 g Sodium: 596mg

KAPAMA DE CHICKEN

Time to Prepare: 10 minutes Time to prepare: 2 hours 4 Servings

Difficulty Average

INGREDIENTS:

f 1 chopped (32-ounce) can tomatoes, drained

f 14 cup dry white wine f 2 tablespoons tomato paste f 3 tablespoons extra-virgin olive oil f 14 teaspoon red pepper flakes f 1 teaspoon ground allspice f 12 teaspoon dried oregano f 2 whole cloves f 1 cinnamon stick f 12 teaspoon sea salt f 1/8 teaspoon freshly ground black pepper DIRECTIONS:

In a large pot, whisk together the tomatoes, wine, tomato paste, olive oil, red pepper flakes, allspice, oregano, cloves, cinnamon stick, sea salt, and pepper. Bring the mixture to a low simmer, stirring occasionally. Allow 30 minutes to simmer, stirring occasionally. Allow the sauce to cool before removing the whole cloves and cinnamon stick.

Preheat oven to 350 degrees Fahrenheit. Place the chicken in a baking dish that measures 9 by 13 inches. Cover the pan with foil and pour the sauce over the chicken. Bake until the internal temperature reaches 165°F.

Calories (per 100g): 220 11g Carbohydrates, 3g Fat 923mg Sodium, 8g Protein

Chapter Four

CHICKEN BREASTS WITH SPINACH AND FETA STUFFING

Time to Prepare: 10 minutes Time to cook: 45 minutes 4 Servings

Difficulty INGREDIENTS:

1 pound fresh baby spinach f 3 minced garlic cloves f 1 lemon zest f 12 teaspoon sea salt f 1/8 teaspoon freshly ground black pepper f 12 cup crumbled feta cheese f 4 boneless, skinless chicken breasts

DIRECTIONS:

Preheat oven to 350 degrees Fahrenheit. Cook the olive oil until it shimmers over medium heat. Mix in the spinach.

Cook, stirring constantly, until the spinach is wilted.

Combine the garlic, lemon zest, salt, and pepper in a mixing bowl. Cook for 30 seconds, constantly stirring.

Allow to cool slightly before mixing in the cheese.

Roll the chicken breasts around the spinach and cheese mixture in an even layer. Using toothpicks or butcher's twine, close the bag. Bake the chicken breasts for 30 to 40 minutes, or until they reach an internal temperature of 165°F, in a 9-by-13-inch baking dish.

Remove from oven and cool for 5 minutes before slicing and serving.

Nutritional Information (per 100g): Calories 263 7g Carbohydrates, 3g Fat 639mg sodium, 17g protein

ROSEMARY BAKED CHICKEN DRUMSTICKS

Time to Prepare: 5 minutes 1 hour to prepare 6 Servings

Difficulty Easy

INGREDIENTS:

f 2 tablespoons chopped fresh rosemary leaves\sf 1 teaspoon garlic powder\sf ½ teaspoon sea salt\sf 1/8 teaspoon freshly ground black pepper\sf Zest of 1 lemon\sf 12 chicken drumsticks

DIRECTIONS:

Preheat oven to 350 degrees Fahrenheit. Mix the rosemary, garlic powder, sea salt, pepper, and lemon zest.

Situate the drumsticks in a 9-by-13-inch baking dish and sprinkle with the rosemary mixture. Bake until the chicken reaches an internal temperature of 165°F.

Nutritional Information (per 100g): 163 Calories 2g Carbohydrates/1g Fat 26g Protein 633mg Sodium

CHICKEN WITH ONIONS, POTATOES, FIGS, AND CARROTS

Time to Prepare: 5 minutes Time to cook: 45 minutes 4 Servings

Level of Difficulty: Moderate

INGREDIENTS:\sf 2 cups fingerling potatoes, halved\sf 4 fresh figs, quartered\sf 2 carrots, julienned\sf 2 tablespoons extra-virgin olive oil\sf 1 teaspoon sea salt, divided\sf ¼ teaspoon freshly ground black pepper\sf 4 chicken leg-thigh quarters\sf 2 tablespoons chopped fresh parsley leaves

DIRECTIONS:

Preheat the oven to 425°F. In a small bowl, toss the potatoes, figs, and carrots with the olive oil, ½ teaspoon of sea salt, and the pepper. Spread in a 9-by-13-inch baking dish.

Season the chicken with the rest of t sea salt. Place it on top of the vegetables. Bake until the vegetables are soft and the chicken reaches an internal temperature of 165°F. Sprinkle with the parsley and serve. Nutritional Information (per 100g):

CHICKEN BREASTS WITH SPINACH AND FETA STUFFING 51

429 Calories 4g Fat 27g Carbohydrates 52g Protein 581mg Sodium

CHICKEN GYROS WITH TZATZIKI

15 minutes for preparation Cooking Time : 1 hours and 20 minutes 6 people

INGREDIENTS: INGREDIENTS: DIFFICULTY LEVEL: MEDIUM

f 1-pound ground chicken breast f 1 onion, grated with excess water wrung out f 2 tablespoons dried rosemary f 1 tablespoon dried marjoram f 6 garlic cloves, minced f ½ teaspoon sea salt f ¼ teaspoon freshly ground black pepper f Tzatziki Sauce

DIRECTIONS:

Preheat oven to 350 degrees Fahrenheit (180 degrees Celsius). Mix the chicken, onion, rosemary, marjoram, garlic, sea salt, and pepper

using food processor. Blend until the mixture forms a paste. Alternatively, mix these ingredients in a bowl until well combined (see preparation tip).

Press the mixture into a loaf pan. Bake until it reaches 165 degrees internal temperature. Take out from the oven and let rest for 20 minutes before slicing.

Slice the gyro and spoon the tzatziki sauce over the top.

(per 100g) nutrition: 289 Calories 1g Fat 20g Carbohydrates 50g Protein 622mg Sodium

MOUSSAKA

10 minutes to prepare 45 minutes of cooking time 8 people

Level of Difficulty: Moderate

INGREDIENTS:

f 5 tablespoons extra-virgin olive oil, divided f 1 eggplant, sliced (unpeeled) f 1 onion, chopped f 1 green bell pepper, seeded and chopped f 1-pound ground turkey f 3 garlic cloves, minced f 2 tablespoons tomato paste f 1 (14-ounce) can chopped tomatoes, drained f 1 tablespoon Italian seasoning f 2 teaspoons Worcestershire sauce

f 1 teaspoon dried oregano f ½ teaspoon ground cinnamon f 1 cup unsweetened nonfat plain Greek yogurt f 1 egg, beaten f ¼ teaspoon freshly ground black pepper f ¼ teaspoon ground nutmeg

f ¼ cup grated Parmesan cheese f 2 tablespoons chopped fresh parsley leaves

DIRECTIONS:

Preheat the oven to 400°F. Cook 3 tablespoons of olive oil until it shimmers. Add the eggplant slices and brown for 3 to 4 minutes per side. Transfer to paper towels to drain.

Return the skillet to the heat and pour the remaining 2 tablespoons of olive oil. Add the onion and green bell pepper. Continue cooking until the vegetables are soft. Remove from the pan and set aside.

Pull out the skillet to the heat and stir in the turkey. Cook for about 5 minutes, crumbling with a spoon, until browned. Stir in the garlic and cook for 30 seconds, stirring constantly.

Stir in the tomato paste, tomatoes, Italian seasoning, Worcestershire sauce, oregano, and cinnamon. Place the onion and bell pepper back to the pan. Cook for 5 minutes, stirring. Combine the yogurt, egg, pepper, nutmeg, and cheese.

Arrange half of the meat mixture in a 9-by-13-inch baking dish. Layer with half the eggplant. Add the remaining meat mixture and the remaining eggplant. Spread with the yogurt mixture. Bake until golden brown. Garnish with the parsley and serve.

(per 100g) nutrition: 338 Calories 5g Fat 16g Carbohydrates 28g Protein 569mg Sodium

DIJON AND HERB PORK TENDERLOIN

10 minutes to prepare 30 Minutes of Preparation 6 people

Average Difficulty

INGREDIENTS: f ½ cup fresh Italian parsley leaves, chopped f 3 tablespoons fresh rosemary leaves, chopped f 3 tablespoons fresh thyme leaves, chopped f 3 tablespoons Dijon mustard f 1 tablespoon extra-virgin olive oil f 4 garlic cloves, minced f ½ teaspoon sea salt f ¼ teaspoon freshly ground black pepper f 1 (1½-pound) pork tenderloin DIRECTIONS:

Preheat the oven to 400°F. Blend the parsley, rosemary, thyme, mustard, olive oil, garlic, sea salt, and

pepper. Process for about 30 seconds until smooth. Spread the mixture evenly over the pork and place it on a rimmed baking sheet.

Bake until the meat reaches an internal temperature of 140°F. Pull out from the oven and set aside for 10 minutes before slicing and serving.

(per 100g) nutrition: 393 Calories 3g Fat 5g Carbohydrates 74g Protein 697mg Sodium

STEAK WITH RED WINE–MUSHROOM SAUCE

Preparation Time : minutes plus 8 hours to marinate Cooking Time : 20 minutes

Servings : 4 Difficulty Level : Difficult

INGREDIENTS: For the Marinade and Steak f 1 cup dry red wine f 3 garlic cloves, minced f 2 tablespoons extra-virgin olive oil f 1 tablespoon low-sodium soy sauce f 1 tablespoon dried thyme f 1 teaspoon Dijon mustard f 2 tablespoons extra-virgin olive oil f 1 to 1½ pounds skirt steak, flat iron steak, or tri-tip steak

For the Mushroom Sauce f 2 tablespoons extra-virgin olive oil f 1-pound cremini mushrooms, quartered f ½ teaspoon sea salt f 1 teaspoon dried thyme f 1/8 teaspoon freshly ground black pepper f 2 garlic cloves, minced f 1 cup dry red wine DIRECTIONS: To Make the Marinade and Steak

In a small bowl, whisk the wine, garlic, olive oil, soy sauce, thyme, and mustard. Pour into a resealable bag and add the steak. Refrigerate the steak to marinate for 4 to 8 hours. Remove the steak from the marinade and pat it dry with paper towels.

Cook the olive oil in large pan until it shimmers.

Situate the steak and cook for about 4 minutes per side until deeply browned on each side and the steak reaches an internal temperature of 140°F. Remove the steak from the skillet and put it on a plate tented with aluminum foil to keep warm, while you prepare the mushroom sauce.

When the mushroom sauce is ready, slice the steak against the grain into ½-inch-thick slices.

To Make the Mushroom Sauce

Cook oil in the same skillet over medium-high heat. Add the mushrooms, sea salt, thyme, and pepper. Cook for about 6 minutes, stirring very infrequently, until the mushrooms are browned.

Sauté the garlic. Mix in the wine, and use the side of a wooden spoon to scoop out any browned bits from the bottom of the skillet. Cook until the liquid reduces by half. Serve the mushrooms spooned over the steak. (per 100g) nutrition: 405 Calories 5g Fat 7g Carbohydrates 33g Protein 842mg Sodium

GREEK MEATBALLS

20 minutes of preparation time 25 minutes of cooking time 4 people

Difficulty Average in difficulty.

INGREDIENTS:

f 2 whole-wheat bread slices f 1¼ pounds ground turkey f 1 egg f ¼ cup seasoned whole-wheat bread crumbs

f 3 garlic cloves, minced f ¼ red onion, grated f ¼ cup chopped fresh Italian parsley leaves f 2 tablespoons chopped fresh mint leaves f 2 tablespoons chopped fresh oregano leaves f ½ teaspoon sea salt f ¼ teaspoon freshly ground black pepper

DIRECTIONS:

Preheat oven to 350 degrees Fahrenheit (180 degrees Celsius). Situate parchment paper or aluminum foil onto the baking sheet. Run the bread under water to wet it, and squeeze out any excess. Shred wet bread into small pieces and place it in a medium bowl.

Add the turkey, egg, bread crumbs, garlic, red onion, parsley, mint, oregano, sea salt, and pepper. Make a thorough mixture. Form the mixture into ¼-cup-size balls. Place the meatballs on the prepared sheet and bake for about 25 minutes, or until the internal temperature reaches 165°F.

Nutrition (for 100g): 350 Calories 6g Fat 10g Carbohydrates 42g Protein 842mg Sodium

LAMB WITH STRING BEANS

10 minutes to prepare 1 hour of cooking Servings : 6 Difficulty Level : Difficult

INGREDIENTS: f ¼ cup extra-virgin olive oil, divided f 6 lamb chops, trimmed of extra fat f 1 teaspoon sea salt, divided f ½ teaspoon freshly ground black pepper f 2 tablespoons tomato paste

f 1½ cups hot water f 1-pound green beans, trimmed and halved crosswise f 1 onion, chopped f 2 tomatoes, chopped

DIRECTIONS: Cook 2 tablespoons of olive oil in large skillet until it shimmers. Season the lamb chops with ½ teaspoon

of sea salt and 1/8 teaspoon of pepper. Cook the lamb in the hot oil for about 4 minutes per side until browned on both sides. Situate the meat to a platter and set aside.

Position the skillet back to the heat and put the remaining 2 tablespoons of olive oil. Heat until it shimmers.

In a bowl, melt the tomato paste in the hot water. Add it to the hot skillet along with the green beans, onion, tomatoes, and the remaining ½ teaspoon of sea salt and ¼ teaspoon of pepper. Bring to a simmer, using a spoon's side to scrape browned bits from the bottom of the pan.

Return the lamb chops to the pan. Allow to boil and adjust the heat to medium-low. Simmer for 45 minutes until the beans are soft, adding additional water as needed to adjust the sauce's thickness. Nutrition (for 100g): 439 Calories 4g Fat 10g Carbohydrates 50g Protein 745mg Sodium

CHICKEN IN TOMATO-BALSAMIC PAN SAUCE

10 minutes to prepare 20 minutes of cooking time 4 people

Average Difficulty

INGREDIENTS f 2 (8 oz. or 7 g each) boneless chicken breasts, skinless f ½ tsp. salt f ½ tsp. ground pepper f 3 tbsps. extra-virgin olive oil f ½ c. halved cherry tomatoes f 2 tbsps. sliced shallot f ¼ c. balsamic vinegar f 1 tbsp. minced garlic f 1 tbsp. toasted fennel seeds, crushed f 1 tbsp. butter

DIRECTIONS:

Slice the chicken breasts into 4 pieces and beat them with a mallet till it reaches a thickness of a ¼ inch.

Use ¼ teaspoons of pepper and salt to coat the chicken. Heat two tablespoons of oil in a skillet and keep the heat to a medium. Cook the chicken breasts on both sides for three minutes. Place it to a serving plate and cover it with foil to keep it warm.

Add one tablespoon oil, shallot, and tomatoes in a pan and cook till it softens. Add vinegar and boil the mix till the vinegar gets reduced by half. Put fennel seeds, garlic, salt, and pepper and cook for about four minutes. Pull it out from the heat and stir it with butter. Pour this sauce over chicken and serve.

Nutrition (for 100g): 294 Calories 17g Fat 10g Carbohydrates Protein (two grams) 639mg Sodium

BROWN RICE, FETA, FRESH PEA, AND MINT SALAD

10 minutes to prepare 25 minutes of cooking time Servings : 4 Difficulty Level : Easy

INGREDIENTS:

❖ 2 c. brown rice

❖ 3 c. water ❖ Salt

❖ 5 oz. or 7 g crumbled feta cheese

❖ 2 c. cooked peas

❖ ½ c. chopped mint, fresh

❖ 2 tbsps. olive oil

❖ Salt and pepper

DIRECTIONS:

Place the brown rice, water, and salt into a saucepan over medium heat, cover, and bring to boiling

point. Turn the lower heat and allow it to cook until the water has dissolved and the rice is soft but chewy. Leave to cool completely

Add the feta, peas, mint, olive oil, salt, and pepper to a salad bowl with the cooled rice and toss to combine Serve and enjoy!

(per 100g) nutrition: 613 Calories 2g Fat 45g Carbohydrates 12g Protein 755mg Sodium

WHOLE GRAIN PITA BREAD STUFFED WITH OLIVES AND CHICKPEAS

10 minutes to prepare 20 minutes of cooking time Servings : 2 Difficulty Level : Average

INGREDIENTS: ◆ 2 wholegrain pita pockets

◆ 2 tbsps. olive oil

◆ 2 garlic cloves, chopped ◆ 1 onion, chopped ◆ ½ tsp. cumin

◆ 10 black olives, chopped ◆ 2 c. cooked chickpeas

◆ Salt and pepper

DIRECTIONS: Slice open the pita pockets and set aside Adjust your heat to medium and set a pan in place.

Add in the

olive oil and heat. Mix in the garlic, onion, and cumin to the hot pan and stir as the onions soften and the cumin is fragrant Add the olives, chickpeas, salt, and pepper and toss everything together until the chickpeas become golden

Set the pan from heat and use your wooden spoon to roughly mash the chickpeas so that some are intact and some are crushed Heat your pita pockets in the microwave, in the oven, or on a clean pan on the stove

Fill them with your chickpea mixture and enjoy!

(per 100g) nutrition: 503 Calories 19g Fat 14g Carbohydrates Protein Content: 7g 798mg Sodium

Chapter Five

ROASTED CARROTS WITH WALNUTS AND CANNELLINI BEANS

10 minutes to prepare 45 minutes of cooking time 4 people

Difficulty Level : Average INGREDIENTS:

f 4 peeled carrots, chopped f 1 c. walnuts f 1 tbsp. honey f 2 tbsps. olive oil f 2 c. canned cannellini beans, drained f 1 fresh thyme sprig f Salt and pepper DIRECTIONS:

Set oven to 400 F/204 C and line a baking tray or roasting pan with baking paper Lay the carrots and walnuts onto the lined tray or pan Sprinkle olive oil and honey over the carrots and walnuts and give everything a rub to make sure each piece is coated Scatter the beans onto the tray and nestle into the carrots and walnuts

Add the thyme and sprinkle everything with salt and pepper Set tray in your oven and roast for about 40 minutes.

Serve and enjoy

(per 100g) nutrition: 385 Calories 27g Fat 6g Carbohydrates 18g Protein 859mg Sodium

SEASONED BUTTERED CHICKEN

10 minutes to prepare 25 minutes of cooking time 4 people

Average Difficulty

INGREDIENTS:

� ½ c. Heavy Whipping Cream � 1 tbsp. Salt � ½ c. Bone Broth � 1 tbsp. Pepper � 4 tbsps. Butter

� 4 Chicken Breast Halves

DIRECTIONS:

1. Place cooking pan on your oven over medium heat and add in one tablespoon of butter. Once the butter

is warm and melted, place the chicken in and cook for five minutes on either side. At the end of this time, the chicken should be cooked through and golden; if it is, go ahead and place it on a plate. 2. Next, you are going to add the bone broth into the warm pan. Add heavy whipping cream, salt, and

pepper. Then, leave the pan alone until your sauce begins to simmer. Allow this process to happen for five minutes to let the sauce thicken up.

3. Finally, you are going to add the rest of your butter and the chicken back into the pan. Be sure to use a spoon to place the sauce over your chicken and smother it completely. Serve Nutrition (for 100g): 350 Calories 25g Fat 10g Carbohydrates 25g Protein 869mg Sodium

DOUBLE CHEESY BACON CHICKEN

10 minutes to prepare 30 Minutes of Preparation Servings : 4 Difficulty Easy difficulty.

INGREDIENTS: f 4 oz. or 113 g. Cream Cheese f 1 c. Cheddar Cheese f 8 strips Bacon f Sea salt f Pepper f 2 Garlic cloves, finely chopped f Chicken Breast f 1 tbsp. Bacon Grease or Butter

DIRECTIONS:

1. Ready the oven to 400 F/204 C Slice the chicken breasts in half to make them thin 2. Season with salt, pepper, and garlic Grease a baking pan with butter and place chicken breasts into it.

Add the cream cheese and cheddar cheese on top of the breasts 3. Add bacon slices as well Place the pan to the oven for 30 minutes Serve hot

(per 100g) nutrition: 610 Calories 32g Fat 3g Carbohydrates 38g Protein 759mg Sodium

SHRIMPS WITH LEMON AND PEPPER

10 minutes to prepare 10 Minutes of Preparation Servings : 4 Difficulty Easy difficulty.

INGREDIENTS: f 40 deveined shrimps, peeled f 6 minced garlic cloves f Salt and black pepper f 3 tbsps. olive oil f ¼ tsp. sweet paprika f A pinch crushed red pepper flake f ¼ tsp. grated lemon zest f 3 tbsps. Sherry or another wine f 1½ tbsps. sliced chives f Juice of 1 lemon DIRECTIONS: Adjust your heat to medium-high and set a pan in place.

Add oil and shrimp, sprinkle with pepper and salt and cook for 1 minute Add paprika, garlic and pepper

flakes, stir and cook for 1 minute. Gently stir in sherry and allow to cook for an extra minute 3. Take shrimp off the heat, add chives and lemon zest, stir and transfer shrimp to plates. Add lemon juice all over and serve

(per 100g) nutrition: 140 Calories 5g Carbohydrates 1 g Fat 18g Protein Sodium 694mg

BREADED AND SPICED HALIBUT Preparation Time : 5 minutes 25 minutes of cooking time 4 people

Difficulty Easy difficulty.

INGREDIENTS:

f ¼ c. chopped fresh chives f ¼ c. chopped fresh dill f ¼ tsp. ground black pepper f ¾ c. panko breadcrumbs f 1 tbsp. extra-virgin olive oil f 1 tsp. finely grated lemon zest f 1 tsp.

sea salt f 1/3 c. chopped fresh parsley f 4 (6 oz. or 170 g. each) halibut fillets

DIRECTIONS:

In a medium bowl, mix olive oil and the rest ingredients except halibut fillets and breadcrumbs

Place halibut fillets into the mixture and marinate for 30 minutes Preheat your oven to 400 F/204 C Set a foil to a baking sheet, grease with cooking spray Dip the fillets to the breadcrumbs and put to the baking sheet Cook in the oven for 20 minutes Serve hot Nutrition (for 100g): 667 Calories 5g Fat 2g Carbohydrates 8g Protein 756mg Sodium

CURRY SALMON WITH MUSTARD

10 minutes to prepare 20 minutes of cooking time Servings : 4 Difficulty Easy difficulty.

INGREDIENTS: f ¼ tsp. ground red pepper or chili powder

f ¼ tsp. turmeric, ground f ¼ tsp. salt f 1 tsp. honey f ¼ tsp. garlic powder

f 2 tsps. whole grain mustard f 4 (6 oz. or 170 g. each) salmon fillets

DIRECTIONS:

1. In a bowl mix mustard and the rest ingredients except salmon Preheat the oven to 350 F/176 C Grease a

baking dish with cooking spray. Place salmon on baking dish with skin side down and spread evenly mustard mixture on top of fillets Place into the oven and cook for 10-15 minutes or until flaky (per 100g) nutrition: 324 Calories 3g Carbohydrates, 9g Fat 34g Protein Sodium 593mg

WALNUT-ROSEMARY CRUSTED SALMON

10 minutes to prepare 25 minutes of cooking time Servings : 4 Difficulty Average in difficulty.

INGREDIENTS: f 1 lb. or 450 g. frozen skinless salmon fillet f 2 tsps. Dijon mustard f 1 clove garlic, minced f ¼ tsp. lemon zest f ½ tsp. honey f ½ tsp. kosher salt f 1 tsp. freshly chopped rosemary f 3 tbsps. panko breadcrumbs f ¼ tsp. crushed red pepper f 3 tbsps. chopped walnuts f 2 tsp. extra-virgin olive oil

DIRECTIONS:

Prepare the oven to 420 F/215 C and use parchment paper to line a rimmed baking sheet. In a bowl combine mustard, lemon zest, garlic, lemon juice, honey, rosemary, crushed red pepper, and salt. In another bowl mix walnut, panko, and 1 tsp oil Place parchments paper on the baking sheet and lay the salmon on it

Spread mustard mixture on the fish, and top with the panko mixture. Spray the rest of olive oil lightly on the salmon. Bake for about 10 -12 minutes or until the salmon is being separated by a fork Serve hot

(per 100g) nutrition: 222 Calories 12g Fat 4g Carbohydrates Protein content: 8g 812mg Sodium

QUICK TOMATO SPAGHETTI Preparation Time : 10 minutes 25 minutes of cooking time 4 people

Average Difficulty

INGREDIENTS: f 8 oz. or 7g spaghetti f 3 tbsps. olive oil f 4 garlic cloves, sliced f 1 jalapeno, sliced f 2 c. cherry tomatoes f Salt and pepper f 1 tsp. balsamic vinegar f ½ c. Parmesan, grated DIRECTIONS: Boil a large pot of water on medium flame. Add a pinch of salt and bring to a boil then add the spaghetti.

Allow cooking for 8 minutes. While the pasta cooks, heat the oil in a skillet and add the garlic and jalapeno. Cook for an extra 1 minute then stir in the tomatoes, pepper, and salt.

Cook for 5-7 minutes until the tomatoes' skins burst.

Add the vinegar and remove off heat. Drain spaghetti well and mix it with the tomato sauce. Sprinkle with cheese and serve right away.

(per 100g) nutrition: 298 Calories 5g Fat 5g Carbohydrates 8g Protein 749mg Sodium

CHILI OREGANO BAKED CHEESE

10 minutes to prepare 25 minutes of cooking time Servings : 4 Difficulty Easy difficulty.

INGREDIENTS: f 8 oz. or 7g feta cheese f 4 oz. or 113g mozzarella, crumbled f 1 sliced chili pepper f 1 tsp. dried oregano f 2 tbsps. olive oil DIRECTIONS: 1. Place the feta cheese in a small deep-dish baking pan. Top with the mozzarella then season with pepper

slices and oregano. cover your pan with lid. Bake in the preheated oven at 350 F/176 C for 20 minutes. Serve the cheese and enjoy it.

(per 100g) nutrition: 292 Calories 2g Fat 7g Carbohydrates Protein (two grams) 733mg Sodium

ITALIAN CHICKEN THAT'S SCRATCHED

10 minutes to prepare 30 Minutes of Preparation 4 Servings; Easy Difficulty

4 CHICKEN LEGS (INGREDIENTS)

1 teaspoon basil (dried)

1 tblsp oregano (dried)

seasonings

olive oil, 3 tbsp.

balsamic vinegar, 1 tblsp.

1. Toss the chicken with basil and oregano and season well. Heat up the oil in a skillet. Toss in the chicken.

oil that has been heated Cover the skillet with a lid after each side has cooked for 5 minutes until golden. 2. Reduce the heat to medium and cook the chicken for 10 minutes on one side before flipping and cooking for another 10 minutes, or until crispy. Enjoy the chicken after it has been prepared.

(per 100g) nutrition: calorie count: 262 11g Carbohydrates, 9g Fat 6 oz. Sodium 693mg

IN YOUR POCKET SEA BASS

10 minutes to prepare 25 minutes of cooking time 4 people

Average Difficulty

INGREDIENTS: 4 sea bass fillets, 4 sliced garlic cloves, 1 sliced celery stalk, 1 sliced zucchini, 1 c. halved cherry tomatoes, halved, 1 shallot, sliced seasonings In a large mixing bowl, combine the garlic, celery, zucchini, tomatoes, shallot, and oregano. To taste, season with salt and pepper.

Place four baking sheets on your work surface. Fill each sheet halfway with the vegetable mixture.

Wrap the paper around the fish fillet to make it look like a pocket. Cook the wrapped fish for 15 minutes in a 350 F/176 C preheated oven. Warm and fresh fish is served.

149 calories per 100g 2g Carbohydrates and 8g Fat 696mg sodium 2g protein

ROASTED CARROTS WITH WALNUTS AND CANNELLINI BEANS

5 MINUTE PREPATION TIME FOR CREAMY SMOKED SALMON PASTA 35-minute preparation time 4 Servings; Moderate Difficulty

INGREDIENTS: f 2 tablespoons olive oil f 2 chopped garlic cloves f 1 shallot, chopped f 4 oz. or 113 g smoked chopped salmon f 1 cup green peas f 1 cup heavy cream f 1 pinch chili flakes (salt and pepper)

6 c. water f 8 oz. or 230 g penne pasta DIRECTIONS: Melt the butter in a large skillet over medium-high heat. Garlic and shallot should be added now. Cook for 5 minutes, or until desired consistency is achieved.

softened. Peas, salt, pepper, and chili flakes should all be added at this point. ten minutes to cook

Cook for another 5-7 minutes with the salmon. Cook for an additional 5 minutes after adding the heavy cream.

Meanwhile, bring a large pot of water to a boil, then add the penne pasta and cook for 8-10 minutes, or until softened. Drain the pasta and combine it with the salmon sauce before serving. (per 100g) nutrition: calorie count: 393 Carbohydrates: 38g Fat: 8g 836mg sodium, 3g protein

CHICKEN WITH GREEK INGREDIENTS IN A SLOW COOKER

20 minutes of preparation time 3 Hours of Preparation 4 Servings; Moderate Difficulty

2 pounds boneless, skinless chicken breasts INGREDIENTS: 1 tablespoon extra-virgin olive oil 12 teaspoon kosher salt, 14 teaspoon black pepper, 1 (12-ounce) jar roasted red peppers, 1 cup Kalamata olives, 1 medium red onion, cut into chunks, 3 tablespoons red wine vinegar, 1 tablespoon minced garlic, 1 teaspoon honey, 1 teaspoon dried oregano, 1 teaspoon dried thyme, 12 cup feta cheese

f basil, parsley, or thyme, chopped

DIRECTIONS:

Cooking spray or olive oil can be used to coat the slow cooker. In a large skillet, warm the olive oil. The chicken breasts should be season on both sides. Sear the chicken breasts on both sides once the oil is hot.

Transfer it to a slow cooker once it's done cooking. Toss the chicken breasts with the red peppers, olives, and onion. Instead of directly on top of the chicken, try to arrange the vegetables around it.

Toss the vinegar, garlic, honey, oregano, and thyme together in a small mixing bowl. Pour it over the chicken once it's all mixed up. Cook for 3 hours on low, or until the chicken is no longer pink in the center. Toss with fresh herbs and crumbled feta cheese.

(per 100g) nutrition: calorie count: 399 Carbohydrates: 12 g (17 g fat) Sodium: 793mg/50g protein

GYROS WITH CHICKEN

10 minutes to prepare 4 Hours of Preparation 4 people

Average Difficulty

2 lbs boneless chicken breasts or chicken tenders INGREDIENTS: 12 cup Greek yogurt f 2 teaspoons dried oregano f 2–4 teaspoons Greek seasoning f 12 small red onion, chopped f 1 lemon's juice f 3 garlic cloves f 2 teaspoons red wine vinegar f 2–3 tablespoons olive oil f 12 cup Greek yogurt f 2 teaspoons dried oregano f 2–4 teaspoons Greek seasoning 1 cup plain Greek yogurt f 1 tablespoon dill weed f 2 tablespoons dill weed f Tzatziki Sauce f 1 small chopped English cucumber 1 teaspoon onion powder a pinch of salt and pepper f f f f f f f f f f Cucumbers f Tomatoes red onion (chopped) feta cheese in diced form f Pita bread, shredded

Cut the chicken breasts into cubes and put them in the slow cooker. Lemon juice, garlic, vinegar, and salt and pepper to taste

Stir to combine the olive oil, Greek yogurt, oregano, Greek seasoning, red onion, and dill in the slow cooker.

5–6 hours on low, 2–3 hours on high Meanwhile, whisk together all of the tzatziki sauce ingredients. Refrigerate until the chicken is done, once everything is well combined.

When the chicken has finished cooking, serve with pita bread and any or all of the toppings listed above. (per 100g) nutrition: 317 Calories 4g Fat 1g Carbohydrates 6g Protein 476mg Sodium

SLOW COOKER CHICKEN CASSOULET

10 minutes to prepare 20 minutes of cooking time Servings : 16

Difficulty Average in difficulty.

INGREDIENTS:

f 1 cup dry navy beans, soaked\sf 8 bone-in skinless chicken thighs

f 1 Polish sausage, cooked and chopped into bite-sized pieces (optional) (optional)

f 1¼ cup tomato juice\sf 1 (28-ounce) can halved tomatoes\sf 1 tbsp Worcestershire sauce

f 1 tsp instant beef or chicken bouillon granules\sf ½ tsp dried basil\sf ½ teaspoon dried oregano\sf ½ teaspoon paprika f ½ cup chopped celery f ½ cup chopped carrot f ½ cup chopped onion DIRECTIONS:

Brush the slow cooker with olive oil or nonstick cooking spray. In a mixing bowl, stir together the tomato juice, tomatoes, Worcestershire sauce, beef bouillon, basil, oregano, and paprika. Make sure the ingredients are well combined.

Place the chicken and sausage into the slow cooker and cover with the tomato juice mixture. Top with celery, carrot, and onion. Cook on low for 10–12 hours.

(per 100g) nutrition: calorie count: 244 7g Fat 25g Carbohydrates 21g Protein 736mg Sodium

SLOW COOKER CHICKEN PROVENCAL\sPreparation Time : 5 minutes Cooking Time : 8 hours Servings : 4\sDifficulty Easy difficulty.

INGREDIENTS:\sf 4 (6-ounce) skinless bone-in chicken breast halves\sf 2 teaspoons dried basil f 1 teaspoon dried thyme f 1/8 teaspoon salt\sf 1/8 teaspoon freshly ground black pepper\sf 1 yellow pepper, diced\sf 1 red pepper, diced\sf 1 (5-ounce) can cannellini beans\sf 1 (5-ounce) can petite tomatoes with basil, garlic, and oregano, undrained\sDIRECTIONS:

1. Brush the slow cooker with nonstick olive oil. Add all the ingredients to the slow cooker and stir to combine. Cook on low for 8 hours.

(per 100g) nutrition: 304 Calories 5g Fat 3g Carbohydrates Protein (four grams) 639mg Sodium

GREEK STYLE TURKEY ROAST

20 minutes of preparation time Cooking Time : 7 hours and 30 minutes 8 Servings; Moderate Difficulty

INGREDIENTS:\sf 1 (4-pound) boneless turkey breast, trimmed\sf ½ cup chicken broth, divided\sf 2 tablespoons fresh lemon juice\sf 2 cups chopped onion\sf ½ cup pitted Kalamata olives\sf ½ cup oil-packed sun-dried tomatoes, thinly sliced\sf 1 teaspoon Greek seasoning\sf ½ teaspoon salt\sf ¼ teaspoon fresh ground black pepper\sf 3 tablespoons all-purpose flour (or whole wheat) (or whole wheat)

DIRECTIONS:\sBrush the slow cooker with nonstick cooking spray or olive oil. Add the turkey, ¼ cup of the chicken

broth, lemon juice, onion, olives, sun-dried tomatoes, Greek seasoning, salt and pepper to the slow cooker.

Cook on low for 7 hours. Scourge the flour into the remaining ¼ cup of chicken broth, then stir gently into the slow cooker. Cook for an additional 30 minutes.

(per 100g) nutrition: 341 Calories 19g Fat 12g Carbohydrates 4g Protein 639mg Sodium

GARLIC CHICKEN WITH COUSCOUS

Preparation Time : 25 minutes Cooking Time : 7 hours 4 Servings; Moderate Difficulty

INGREDIENTS:\sf 1 whole chicken, cut into pieces f 1 tablespoon extra-virgin olive oil f 6 cloves garlic, halved\sf 1 cup dry white wine\sf 1 cup couscous\sf ½ teaspoon salt\sf ½ teaspoon pepper\sf 1 medium onion, thinly sliced\sf

2 teaspoons dried thyme f 1/3 cup whole wheat flour DIRECTIONS:\s1. Cook the olive oil in a heavy skillet. When skillet is hot, add the chicken to sear. Make sure the chicken

pieces don't touch each other. Cook with the skin side down for about 3 minutes or until browned. 2. Brush your slow cooker with nonstick cooking spray or olive oil. Put the onion, garlic, and thyme into\sthe slow cooker and sprinkle with salt and pepper. Stir in the chicken on top of the onions. 3. In a separate bowl, whisk the flour into the wine until there are no lumps, then pour over the chicken. Cook on low for 7 hours or until done. You can cook on high for 3 hours as well. Serve the chicken over\sthe cooked couscous and spoon sauce over the top.

(per 100g) nutrition: 440 Calories 5g Fat 14g Carbohydrates 8g Protein 674mg Sodium

CHICKEN KARAHI

5 minutes of preparation time Cooking Time : 5 hours Servings : 4\sDifficulty Easy difficulty.

INGREDIENTS:\sf 2 lbs. chicken breasts or thighs\sf ¼ cup olive oil\sf 1 small can tomato paste\sf 1 tablespoon butter\sf 1 large onion, diced\sf ½ cup plain Greek yogurt\sf ½ cup water\sf 2 tablespoons ginger in garlic paste\sf 3 tablespoons fenugreek leaves\sf 1 teaspoon ground coriander\sf 1 medium tomato f 1 teaspoon red chili f 2 green chilies\sf 1 teaspoon turmeric\sf 1 tablespoon garam masala f 1 teaspoon cumin powder f 1 teaspoon sea salt\sf ¼ teaspoon nutmeg

DIRECTIONS:\sBrush the slow cooker with nonstick cooking spray. In a small bowl, thoroughly mix all of the spices.

Mix in the chicken to the slow cooker, followed by the ingredients' rest, including the spice mixture. Stir until everything is well mixed with the spices.

Cook on low for 4–5 hours. Serve with naan or Italian bread.

(per 100g) nutrition: 345 Calories 9g Fat 10g Carbohydrates Protein Content: 7g 715mg Sodium